KISS YOUR ASH GOOD-BYE!

AMERICA'S #1 STOP SMOKING GUIDEBOOK

A Psychologist's Step-by-Step Guide for Quitting Smoking Forever!

Joel D. Block, Ph.D., ABPP

CONTENTS

I. INTRODUCTION

1. So you think maybe you want to stop smoking?

It's really a great idea! It is not an exaggeration to say that if you successfully stop smoking, it would be about the most important thing you could do for yourself these days. Don't fool yourself: there is no longer any question about it – smoking is one of the most destructive things we do to ourselves. And stopping always provides benefits, no matter how little or how long you've smoked.

Note: Throughout this guide the term "Smoking" may be actual smoking or it may equally be a nicotine product being referred to. The distinction is not critical. In either case, the tips, suggestions and guidelines remain the same. In other words, this manual is applicable with the assistance of nicotine products or without them.

2. Do you "have enough motivation"?

Motivation is a complicated issue, but be careful not to use this question against yourself. Most everyone who thinks about stopping smoking "has enough motivation," but maybe has not been able to get it all working together to lead to quickly and easily stopping. If you're like most smokers, part of you would very much like to stop smoking (otherwise you wouldn't be reading this), but another part of you would very much like to continue smoking (otherwise you would have stopped already). Usually, the balance between these two tendencies fluctuates a lot. What these pages attempt is to help you boost the "want-to-stop" side just long enough and steadily enough so that you can break the chain around your neck and be free to make a calm and easy decision later.

A lot of people ask this motivation question because they really feel they should wait until some time in their life when they will have a super-dose of "motivation." In this way they can forever put off stopping. Don't let this happen to you, because you could wait forever. You "do have enough motivation" to work with right now.

3. Why is stopping smoking so difficult?

The intricacies of your having become dependent on cigarettes will be discussed in detail later, as a means of explaining how to break the dependency. For now, a general psychological/physical understanding will suffice.

Whether or not you enjoy the *taste* of cigarettes, you clearly get something out of smoking, or else you wouldn't continue to smoke. Indeed, the rewards, or reinforcements, for smoking are consistent and immediate. There is, of course, the nicotine hit. Nicotine is potent but so is the habit of smoking—that's why the various nicotine products alone aren't nearly fully successful. Each time you light a cigarette, you are rewarded with any number of possible reinforcements: reduction of tension, alleviation of anxiety, a sense of well-being, good taste, and alleviation of feelings of boredom. Then there is the elimination of awkwardness from having nothing to do with your hands and for some, a temporary distancing between yourself and others. What's more, these occur as soon as you light up.

The negative consequences of smoking, on the other hand, are neither immediate nor consistent, even though they are definitely more significant in the long run. An elevated *overall* anxiety level, massive assaults on your body systems, significantly increased risk of many major debilitating and terminal diseases, and even regular annoying symptoms are consequences which are neither consistent nor immediate. Some of them you get used to (shortness of breath, coughing), some you aren't aware of (significantly elevated heart rate and blood pressure). Some you can't be sure will ever happen to you (cancer, emphysema, coronary artery disease), and others happen hours after you smoke (coughing up phlegm in the morning).

In a conditioning sense, reinforcements must be immediate and consistent to be effective. If you coughed up phlegm for five minutes immediately after each cigarette, you would readily be conditioned to stop smoking automatically.

As you can see, the balance, in a behavioral conditioning sense, is on the side of continuing to smoke. To combat and defeat this imbalance, what is required is a cognitive understanding of what is happening and what consequences really are the more important ones in the long run. Also required is a conscious, active, and sustained effort to stop, bringing to the fore other behavioral science mechanisms which will make not smoking eventually become automatic, following an initial "despite-yourself" effort.

4. How important is finding the right "technique" to stop?

So many people who want to stop smoking have spent so many years of their lives trying out so many techniques to stop smoking! This is because they believe that once they find "the right technique," they will be able to sit back and let their technique do the work for them. It's not going to happen. Techniques and tips do matter, but they aren't everything. Unless you've thought out your decision to stop well, cleared away your own mental obstacles to quitting, and gone into it with the right attitude, no technique will work. You'll quit quitting before you quit smoking!

5. How can you have "the right attitude"?

a. <u>Confront the part of you that is hoping for magic.</u>

If you're like most smokers, you might deep down hope either that someday you'll just wake up and find that you don't want to smoke anymore or that some technique of stopping will instantly make you never have an urge to smoke again. Forget it! First of all, it hasn't happened yet, right? Second, there's no reason to expect it will happen, because smoking has been such an important part of your life. And finally, how many people do you think would still be smoking if a "magic cure" had been discovered?

b. <u>Stop smoking for yourself—or for someone you love dearly.</u>

If you feel that your quitting is something you're doing for your doctor or someone not central to your life, you're likely to have trouble. Stopping smoking is difficult and requires a lot of commitment. Chances are that the only persons you feel enough of this commitment toward are yourself or someone who means the world to you. Your children, a husband or wife or some other loved one will work. I lost my father before the age of four; I didn't want my children to have the same experience. That helped me in my effort to quit enormously. That's because, even if I didn't care enough about myself, my children's well-being meant everything. So, if it not for yourself, it must be someone who is very important to you. Someone you feel indebted to. Of course, you must also remind yourself that *you* will benefit enormously by not smoking!

c. <u>Choose a positive focus, not a negative one.</u>

When you stop smoking, you are taking something important out of your life. Smoking definitely gives you pleasure and a nicotine boost, although this pleasure and boost is different for different people and may have nothing to do with "taste." Even if you don't "enjoy" many cigarettes, you obviously get *something* out of them or else you wouldn't smoke them. Therefore, it *is* a deprivation to give up cigarettes. Nicotine is addictive!

On the other hand (and this side of the coin is just as true), when you stop smoking, you are giving yourself something terribly valuable. This could be immediate reduction of smoking-related symptoms, a likelihood of living a longer and healthier life, or just a chance to accomplish something, to finally get this load off your back, a load which has troubled you for some time. Whatever it is in your particular case, it certainly is true that stopping smoking will *give* you something.

Now, when you stop, it is strictly your choice as to which of these sides you choose to focus on. You could feel sorry for yourself, feel deprived, and dwell on how great a sacrifice you are making. Or, you could focus your thoughts instead on what you are doing *for* yourself, what you are giving *to* yourself. In my experience, I have found that people who adopt a positive focus have an easier time quitting and feel less deprived while stopping.

d. <u>Confront the part of yourself that thinks you cannot quit.</u>

There is no one who *cannot* quit smoking! Think about it – if you were locked up without cigarettes for a week, you'd survive. If someone could offer you millions of dollars (or something you perhaps value more) to stop smoking, you would do it. You clearly have the capacity to quit; it's just that you haven't, up until now, been willing to endure the "pain" you expect to feel when you decide not to put another cigarette into your mouth. This distinction is important: you are dealing with a choice that you *can* make (but haven't wanted to), not with something that is impossible.

Many people strongly hold on to the belief that they cannot quit because in this way they can be at peace with themselves. If you think you can't possibly stop doing something, you don't have to feel bad because you continue to do it. The fact is that multi-millions of Americans have quit smoking, some with ease, but many with considerable difficulty. With the help of the guidelines given here, you can do it too, and probably without such great difficulty.

e. <u>Commit yourself firmly and optimistically to whatever goals you set.</u>

In stopping smoking, you have complete predictive control over outcome. If you believe you won't be able to make it, you certainly won't. If you believe you'll succeed, you definitely will. This is quite a remarkable thing – and is the closest thing to magic I've ever come across. Let's look at it in more detail.

When you are in a no-smoking area, which is quite common these days, you probably don't smoke *and* find it easy not to. Once you have accepted the idea that you are not going to smoke, not only do you not smoke, but it's also not difficult. This principle can be put to use for whatever goals you set. Imagine you make a commitment to yourself, for example, not to smoke at a party. If this is a very strong commitment (such as when you say to yourself, "I will not smoke at this party *no matter what*: if I'm suffering too much, I'll leave and take a walk, or I'll go to a movie, or I'll sit and eat for three solid hours," or whatever), not only does this become a self-fulfilling prophecy (you won't smoke), but also it becomes surprisingly easy and you'll never have to resort to the extreme escapes you mentioned. If, on the other hand, you go in saying to yourself, "I'll try not to smoke at this party, but I'll probably give in after a couple of hours at the most," you can expect to struggle all the way and will almost certainly, like clockwork, light up two hours after you arrive. What you decide you are able to do is, in fact, what you will be able to do.

How can we understand this direct relationship between the strength of your commitment and the amount of discomfort or pain you'll experience? Psychologists can only speculate, but it seems that a great part of the "pain" that we feel as an urge to smoke, despite the nicotine withdrawal, is just the anxiety involved in making a decision. Decision-making in itself is a painful process. Someone who is trying to quit smoking, even with the assistance of a nicotine product, but who has not committed himself to any goal, must face a new decision (do I smoke a cigarette now or not?) every time he gets an urge to smoke. If he has, instead, made a non-negotiable decision (for two hours, two days, two months, or forever) not to smoke, he can avoid this recurring "decision anxiety."

Practically (and this is the most useful "tip" one can get), this means you should do whatever you can to "psych" yourself up to be fully committed and optimistic about following through on whatever plan you adopt, be it to avoid one cigarette, cut down, quit for a month, or quit for good. In case you were wondering, those people who could somehow one day throw away their cigarettes and not suffer with never smoking again are always those who made a "no matter what" commitment to themselves. They didn't torment themselves with deliberation.

II. GETTING OFF

There are two parts to the stop smoking process. You should come to see them as two different concerns. The first is getting off and the second is staying off. You may be someone, or you undoubtedly know someone, who has stopped smoking for some period of time, only to start up again. Given how hard it is to stop, and how relatively easy it is to stay off once you've stopped, this is really a tragedy – and it can easily be avoided.

Because these are separate tasks, this book is divided into two sections: Getting Off and Staying Off. It is crucial that you take these jobs one at a time. A common cause of defeat is when people say to themselves, "I know I can get off, but since I think I won't be able to stay off, I won't even bother to stop in the first place".

It's hard enough to first get off cigarettes without carrying the extra burden of worrying about the whole rest of your life too. You'd never be able to get out of bed in the morning if you made yourself worry about all the difficulties you will have to face for the rest of your life. Take the stop smoking challenge in small, manageable pieces. You'll better be able to handle the later phases once you've mastered the earlier ones. With your resources, any help you may get here or from others or with the assistance of a temporary nicotine delivery method, and with some initial success under your belt, the long-term will be very easy to take care of.

There will be more about staying off later. For now, just focus on the very beginning of stopping.

6. What should you know about techniques?

We can profitably go on now to talk more of techniques, but remember that techniques don't "work" unless:

1) you realize there's no magic,
2) you're stopping for yourself and/or someone you love dearly,
3) you feel you are giving yourself something if you stop smoking.
4) you believe you can quit, and
5) you firmly plan to stick to whatever plan of action you choose, and you believe you'll be able to implement and stick to the plan.

The way most plans to stop smoking are classified is to say whether they are "tapering off" plans or "cold turkey" plans. Actually, the distinction is sort of phony, because everyone who stops eventually goes "cold turkey," although he/she may or may not cut down in preparation for this event. In line with my direct approach, I must clearly point out the hard facts (even though they may be obvious): If you plan to quit your smoking habit (whatever the technique you use), this means that one day you will *stop smoking*. Techniques and tips are always aimed at preparing you for this day and helping you cope with what follows it, but never eliminates its eventual occurrence.

7. Tapering down: good or bad?

Many people do well by tapering down as a preparation for stopping – mainly because it demonstrates that it *is* possible to change smoking patterns, because it isn't so frightening not to smoke for a while when you know you'll be able to smoke again soon, and because it provides a preparation period before what seems to be so drastic – stopping altogether.

Still, many people have negative experiences with tapering down. Many people report, after they eventually stop smoking, that their tapering down period was useful or necessary, but that it was even more difficult to do than to stop altogether. A more common bad experience with tapering down is that the plan somehow is "ditched" before the end is reached.

What can you learn from these experiences? First, it must be understood that tapering down does not, in itself, lead to automatic quitting, in the sense of: the fewer you smoke, the less you want to smoke. Many people give up in their attempt to gradually taper down to zero because they are disappointed to find that their desire to smoke doesn't simultaneously taper down to zero and they decide something must not be working right. Actually, this is typical –because even when you taper down, the final act of quitting still always involves a big jump.

Indeed, tapering down is so often difficult because the opposite occurs: the less you smoke, the *more* you want to smoke. Think of it this way – when you taper down, you end up watching the clock, waiting for the next cigarette, anticipating it, imagining how great it will taste, building up a stronger need to smoke, perhaps feeling uncomfortable because you aren't smoking. Then you light that delightful cigarette, and it does taste good and it makes you feel better immediately. In psychological terms, you are arranging it so that each individual cigarette is even more rewarding than when you smoked normally. This sets up a tremendous imbalance: you are smoking fewer cigarettes, but increasing your desire for cigarettes. This imbalance will tend to make you want to go either way – to decide to quit completely or to go back up to your usual rate or even higher.

To summarize, tapering down is usually very difficult and is not a pattern many smokers can casually switch into. People can and do taper down, sometimes for even long periods of time, but they must always work at it; it doesn't just automatically maintain itself. Your psyche not only misses the smoking habit, your body misses its usual nicotine ration.

Therefore, a tapering-down period should not last too long. How many times have you or people you know tried to cut down, only to abandon the plan because "something came up"? Because the tapering-down period is unstable and imbalanced, it is very easily disrupted. The longer you take, the greater the chance that that "something" will come up.

Once again, if you decide to taper down in preparation for quitting, because you feel it would be useful to "take the edge" off of the "plunge," only do so with the knowledge that a "plunge" still awaits you and only allow yourself a short period of time (less than, say, two weeks).

8. What about just cutting-down as your final goal?

Many people who are not happy with their smoking would be satisfied if they could cut down to just 3 or 4 cigarettes a day, instead of stopping completely. Indeed, this isn't hard to understand - most of us think that a few cigarettes a day aren't that harmful, don't cost that much, and would probably all be very enjoyable. The only problem is that this is untrue, even a few cigarettes a day are harmful and this goal is unattainable for the vast majority of smokers. In my own experience with hundreds of smokers, I have *never met one* who could taper *down* to this low level and stay there. That includes me!

You really must again and again confront yourself on this issue. The lingering secret hope of many people who fail again and again at quitting is that they will be one of those very, very few people who will be able to just have, for example, one cigarette after each meal. If you fancy that maybe you'll be able to do it, this must be based on a view of yourself that you're really someone super-special, because millions have tried it before and failed.

The reasons for this come straight from the section above: smoking at a lower level is an imbalanced situation and is easily disturbed. Add to that the nicotine hunger and it's not going to work. That's the hard reality.

Perhaps you're thinking right now about a couple of people you know who do smoke only 3 or 4 or no cigarettes a day. I know of some too. But they are *always* people who never smoked more than this regularly. You just don't settle down into a lower level and "automatically" stay there; it takes a lot of work to maintain it and the minute you let up watching it, you work your way back to your usual level. Besides, the research is clear; these people are endangering their health.

9. What kind of tapering down is best?

The most common kind of tapering down, unfortunately, is the worst. This involves watching the clock, waiting a certain amount of time between cigarettes. This is torture. Another common technique involves eliminating cigarettes from successively more and more situations where you usually smoke (for example, no smoking while walking and then also no cigarettes while driving, and later, none with coffee, and so on). This procedure usually is less painful; but is too often done over too long a period of time – and many people then start driving or walking less, for obvious reasons. Or just break the commitment.

One technique that minimizes the problem of making smoking too reinforcing is the one that involves starting smoking later and later each day. If you choose to taper down, I recommend this procedure:

You start smoking tomorrow morning as usual and smoke at your usual rate once you start. The next day, you do not smoke for two hours and then smoke freely the rest of the day. The third day start four hours after getting up, and so on. Once you start smoking, smoke freely. In this way, only the first cigarette you smoke each day will have increased reinforcing value for you. You will note that this timetable involves quitting completely roughly one week from now.

Another reason for preferring this technique is a physical one, which will be explained in more detail in Section 16. Briefly stated, the urge to smoke a cigarette is partly supplied by the physical sensation of "coming down" from the nicotine fix of the cigarette before. Only the first cigarette of the morning doesn't have this additional physical input and is therefore easier to avoid.

10. What are other possible preparations for quitting?

The other possibilities, in terms of number of cigarettes, are obvious. If you don't cut down before stopping, you can either continue to smoke as usual until then or else increase your smoking to prepare you for it. This unusual approach has often proved helpful: you double your smoking for a few days so that, at least in the beginning, it actually becomes a relief to stop smoking.

11. What techniques or tips help people while they aren't smoking?

Here is a list of tips compiled from various sources:

LIST

(1) Temporarily avoid those situations where you are inclined to smoke heavily.
(2) Hide the ashtrays and cigarettes.
(3) Find something to do with your hands.
(4) Use non-caloric mouth-occupiers: dietetic candy and gum, pencils, celery sticks, etc.
(5) Sip from a glass of water all day long.
(6) Use walking around or deep breathing as a substitute pace-breaker.
(7) Deep breathing: take 5 slow *deep* breaths, letting your muscles go more and more limp each time you exhale.
(8) Don't buy more than a pack at a time; never a carton.
(9) Announce your plans to quit to people around you to enhance your commitment.
(10) Change brands regularly.
(11) Indulge yourself in other ways, using the money you're saving or otherwise.
(12) Develop a set of rules about where you can and cannot smoke (e.g., only in the

basement or bathroom, or out of your favorite chair).

(13) Leave your cigarettes in the mailbox or your car so you have to travel to get one.

(14) Keep putting your not-smoking savings in a transparent jar so you can watch your savings grow – then use them for yourself.

(15) Wrap your cigarettes in a large sheet of paper, keeping it in place with a rubber band. Each time you take a cigarette, unwrap the package, record the *time, occasion,* your *mood,* and how *important* the cigarette seems (1 to 5), then rewrap the package. You will find you've cut down significantly just because of the nuisance of wrapping and because of keeping count. You'll learn some interesting things about your patterns of smoking.

(16) Never carry matches or a lighter.

(17) Don't smoke for ½ hour after rising or meals, ½ hour before retiring. Extend this time.

(18) Postpone smoking by making yourself wait until a later time and activity, when you'll again *decide* whether to smoke or postpone once more.

(19) Use "hot" tasting candies or cough drops (or juices with lemon or other peppery spices) to substitute for the burning taste of cigarettes.

(20) Use a plastic cigarette.

(21) Break a fresh filter off a cigarette. Douse it in a strong mouthwash and put in a clean cigarette holder. Use this as a sucking substitute.

(22) Use a cigarette case with a timer.

(23) Draw red lines on your cigarettes, smoking only to the red line. Gradually move the line closer and closer to the tip.

(24) Use mouthwash sprays, mouthwashes, brush your teeth often.

(25) When you first quit, spend many hours in places that do not allow smoking.

(26) Give your cigarettes to someone else so you have to ask for each cigarette.

(27) Collect your butts, store them in a jar half filled with water. Disgust yourself by looking at it or smelling it.

(28) Keep postponing the first cigarette of the day later and later.

(29) Make a bet with someone about your quitting.

(30) Take frequent showers.

(31) Inhale only some puffs on each cigarette instead of every one.

(32) Substitute tea for coffee, if you have a strong coffee/cigarette link.

(33) Quickly leave the table at the end of a meal.

(34) Go to bed earlier, arise later to give yourself less smoking time.

(35) Have your dentist clean your teeth when you first stop; send curtains, quilts to be cleaned to get rid of tobacco traces and discourage yourself from undoing these results.

(36) Quit with a "buddy" and help each other.

(37) Cut out smoking on successively more and more occasions (driving, telephone, drinks, etc.).

(38) Make yourself buy (and throw away most of) a new pack for each cigarette you smoke.

(39) Throw away your expensive lighters, ashtrays, cigarette cases.

(40) Try nicotine-substitute products. These products deliver nicotine through various means—orally, transdermally (patches), nasal (sprays), etc.

Inasmuch as you know yourself best and no technique works for everybody, you should carefully look over this list. Choose the ideas that you think might be useful for you and then try them. If they help, fine; if not, discard them. You probably have heard some other ideas from other people, and even can invent a few of your own.

12. Is it all right to use crutches to help you stop?

Many of the tips above involve doing something artificial to help you not smoke. This is perfectly all right. Some people argue that you should stop without temporary aids because sooner or later you'll have to do without them. For example, they say you should not distance yourself from cigarettes when you first stop, because that's artificial: there will always be cigarettes around. This is true, but it ignores something basic about quitting: the most difficulties and greatest adjustments occur within a couple of weeks of stopping.

To help yourself with whatever crutches you choose for this period is perfectly reasonable. By the time you choose to forego the crutches, you'll be much stronger, with more emotional energy available than when you first quit.

Generally, I advise people to allow themselves *whatever* aids, substitutes, or crutches they think will help – for two full weeks after quitting. On that very day (two weeks from the quitting day), they should plan to give up the aid and return to usual patterns. This works very well, e.g., stop using sucking candies, throwing away the plastic cigarettes, going again to parties, again drinking coffee with breakfast are all very possible on this two-week date.

One man doubted this was true for him. He was convinced that he was able to stop smoking only because of the help of sucking candies. It had gotten so that he was spending nearly as much on candies as he had been on cigarettes. He dreaded the day he'd stop eating so much candy, certain that he'd be forced to smoke again. It was strongly suggested that he go "cold turkey" on the candy for only 24 hours exactly two weeks after he quit smoking. To his tremendous relief, this was extremely easy, even though the candies had been so crucial only two weeks earlier. After all, a two-week habit is all he had developed. The smoking habit was substantially and independently weakened in the meantime, so there was no re-burst of difficulty.

13. What about weight?

As you know, weight gain is a common concern of would-be ex-smokers. While by no means a minor issue, the weight problem is often exaggerated. Roughly speaking, about a quarter of the people who quit smoking lose weight. Another quarter stays roughly the same. Another quarter gain less than four pounds. So three quarters of the people have no weight gain problem at all. There still remains, though, that last quarter who gain more than four pounds. What can be said to alleviate your concern about this happening to you?

First, you should know that your weight gain from stopping smoking will not be a serious health risk, even though the concerns about appearance and fitting into clothes are not so easily dismissed. To do the damage to your heart comparable to that from smoking a pack a day, you would have to gain 80 pounds!

You should also know that many people have been able to turn their concern about weight into a rationalization for justifying their returning to smoking. Many quitters start eating many very fattening foods – some of which they never enjoyed eating before. It's as if they were setting out to gain enough weight so they could go back to smoking with good conscience. I know this was in fact what was happening in these cases, because just getting the knowledge and insight into what was (unconsciously) happening was enough for them to end this self-defeating pattern.

For this reason, and for the reasons given in the preceding section, I encourage you to allow yourself whatever food substitutes for smoking you wish, once again for two weeks. To undercut the irrational use of weight gain, don't weigh yourself for two weeks. Make a deal with yourself that you won't allow yourself to be concerned about weight for two weeks. Or alternatively, set some limit of weight gain (say 5 or 10 pounds) that you tell yourself you'll allow before you start to concentrate on your eating.

Then, if you reach your limit (you probably won't), or when two weeks passes, you'll find it very easy to stop your overeating or change to non-fattening oral substitutes. If not, it is probably because you are setting out to gain weight, albeit unconsciously.

Some people believe that it is possible to gain weight after quitting smoking even without eating more. This is contested by many doctors and, indeed, by far most quitters who gained weight readily agree they did a lot more eating. Even if there is a metabolism change, though, it is likely to be temporary and small. After the two weeks' grace period, it is not unreasonable to expect yourself to adjust your eating habits as necessary.

Finally, some tips to help minimize weight gain[†]:

(1) Use only low-calorie foods for snacking.

(2) Don't take second helpings.

(3) Eat more frequently, but in smaller amounts; have your normal dinner dessert two hours after dinner, etc.

(4) Avoid rich desserts: use fruits for your sweets craving.

(5) Cut calories where you can. Use sugar substitutes, cut down on desserts and drinks.

(6) Find non-edible things to chew or suck on.

(7) Use water as your chief oral substitute.

(8) Get a little more exercise; for example, by walking briskly part of the way to work.

(9) Certain olfactory signals in the form of concentrated vapors (smells) can also be used to decrease the desire to eat

---

[†] Thanks to the New York American Cancer Society.

and trigger anti-hunger responses in the brain. For example, concentrated oils extracted from sour green apples or blends of mint activate the satiety areas of the brain and lead to decreased appetite.

14. What can you expect to happen when you stop?

You will have to deal with two kinds of "problems" when you first stop smoking. One involves unpleasant physical and psychological sensations, which people usually call "withdrawal symptoms." The other involves recurring "urges" to smoke.

There is tremendous variation from person to person in terms of the size of these problems, with many experiencing no withdrawal symptoms and very brief experience of desires to smoke. Moreover, within the same person, there may be big differences in difficulty from one stopping experience to another. So even if you've stopped before, you really cannot be sure that you will have the same experience when you stop now.

A big portion of the rest of this book is aimed at explaining and discussing withdrawal symptoms and urges – so that you will be adequately prepared for them and know how to handle them.

15. What should you know about withdrawal symptoms?

In my experience with many smokers, I have come across an incredible range of withdrawal symptoms. Some people have nose bleeds, some chest pains, and some have tingling fingers. Some cannot sleep well, others sleep all the time. There are headaches, back aches, sore tongues and sore backs. Then there are the more common ones: irritability, tenseness, a feeling of climbing the walls, depression, hunger, and a hard-to-describe loss of ability to concentrate, with a "cottony" feeling in the mouth, along with a feeling that the tongue is thicker.

One hesitates to mention all of these things to people, because we have a strange way of going out and having all the problems we hear about. They are mentioned here, though, to make sure you realize that whatever "strange" reaction you may have is not so strange.

At the same time, you should know that it is possible *not* to have any withdrawal symptoms. Some people are convinced there is no such thing as withdrawal symptoms because they never had any.

a. Withdrawal symptoms are always temporary.

This is the most important thing you should know. I've never heard of any lasting more than three weeks or so unless the person was obsessing about them. For most, withdrawal symptoms are gone by the fourth or fifth day. It's impossible to make completely accurate predictions for you specifically, because each person is different. Still, each cluster of symptoms

seems to have a general time span.
Irritability and difficulties concentrating are usually finished after the first few days.
Increased coughing usually lasts only a couple of days. Sleep disturbances tend to be at the other end, maybe lasting a couple of weeks, and so on.

When I first heard of each of these symptoms, I used to spend hours consulting with doctors, trying to understand and explain to the sufferer what was going on. Most all the symptoms are fairly explainable (for example, you may cough up more phlegm when you stop because your lungs' self-cleaning functions are no longer paralyzed when you stop smoking). Luckily, though, I finally realized that I could stop trying to understand and explain all of them, because by the time I next saw the person having a symptom, it was almost always already gone, without the help of my understanding it.

It is crucial that you understand and believe that whatever problems you have when you stop will soon be finished. People can withstand most any discomfort or pain if they know it will soon end. Otherwise they buckle under, thinking they have only one way to end the suffering. In fact, your withdrawal symptoms will go away if you smoke, *and* they'll go away if you don't smoke.

b. <u>Withdrawal symptoms are understandable.</u>

Are you surprised that you may suffer some discomfort or agitation when you stop smoking? Think about it. When you are a smoker, you do *nothing* as often as smoke, except maybe blink and breathe. A pack-and-a-half smoker smokes more than 10,000 cigarettes a year! This is done year after year and clearly becomes an integral part of your psychological, physical, and social life. Recall nicotine is an addictive drug! Is it any wonder that you experience some disruption or disturbance when you finally stop smoking? It seems to me that people who have withdrawal symptoms shouldn't be surprised; not to have them is much less understandable.

c. <u>Withdrawal symptoms are good.</u>

Sounds perverted? Actually, difficulty when you stop can go a long way toward cementing your success. If you experience memorable discomfort in the beginning, you will find it difficult later to bring yourself to waste your earlier ordeal; you will make certain your suffering was not for naught. People who find it extremely easy to quit will sometimes start smoking again because they can look forward to another easy time quitting again (although they often are wrong).

d. <u>Withdrawal symptoms are bearable.</u>

Perhaps all this talk about suffering is beginning to scare you. You certainly will not have all the difficulties mentioned here. More important, you probably are expecting more trouble than you actually will have.

While it is reasonable for you to anticipate discomforts in the beginning, you almost certainly (if you're like most smokers) expect them to be worse than they actually will be. It always looks worse when it's ahead of you than when it's behind you, but also *while* it's happening it's more bearable than you anticipate.

e. Withdrawal symptoms are often used for rationalizations.

The misuse of the fear of, or experience of, withdrawal symptoms is the main tool of those seeking a way not to stop smoking. The internal thoughts may go something like this: "I'm having a bad headache because of quitting. I could bear it, I suppose, for a while, but I couldn't stand this for the rest of my non-smoking life. I'll give up sometime or other, so why fight it – I might as well give up now." The fallacy here is in the rest-of-my-life business. The headache will disappear soon without taking a cigarette.

Whenever a withdrawal symptom is the basis for going back to smoking, it is always possible to discover the fallacy in reasoning. Generally, the fallacy involves telling yourself: a) the symptom won't go away, b) the difficulty should not be happening – that something must be going wrong, c) your suffering will interfere with successful abstinence, or d) you won't be able to bear the hurt. These points were covered in the preceding four sections; make certain you agree that the rationalizations given here are unfounded and are just some of the many brilliant ways we humans are so able to make our thoughts serve our continuing to smoke.

16. Do these symptoms imply that nicotine is addictive?

Yes, of course, but that's not the whole story. There are also powerful psychological factors or else nicotine delivery systems (the patch, pill, gum, etc.) would be 100% effective and they are not. To understand this, consider heroin. Heroin is clearly addictive. Yet, heroin addicts end their physical addiction in that initial period of "cold turkey," when they no longer physically rely on heroin. As you know, this is not the end for most of them and many return again to the drug – now for other, non-physical reasons. Just like cigarette smokers who go back to smoking after quitting, it is also for non-physical reasons. Researchers agree that the physical addiction part of cigarette smoking ends within a few days time after stopping, when the nicotine has left the system. If you have an addiction to nicotine, you break it by not smoking for just a few days. Clearly the psychological issues involved in your smoking are important ones to be concerned about.

"Withdrawal symptoms," as mentioned above, are physical and psychological, and last more than one day. From the physical perspective, nicotine is a strong chemical. In fact, it is poisonous. If you inject one drop of nicotine in your bloodstream, it would kill you instantly. Obviously, you don't get enough nicotine in the smoke of one cigarette to kill you. But you do get enough to mobilize your body's defenses against the intrusion of a harmful substance. Your blood pressure and heart rate increase, you make your adrenalin flow quickly, all working to fight off the "intruder." It is these involuntary physical responses of the body that can contribute to the chronic diseases that often result from smoking. One startling fact should be mentioned here: nicotine *is so poisonous* that you would die a few hours after just one cigarette if somehow your body's defense system weren't working. If you try to hold your hand steady while smoking, you'll be able to see that you are less and less steady with each drag on a cigarette. In a sense, then, by smoking you are giving yourself many "highs" a day. Your system gets used to this stimulation, and you miss it when you first stop smoking. In fact, even while smoking, these physical results of smoking make you want to smoke. The "coming down" from the cigarette you smoked half an hour ago can stimulate an urge to smoke now. This is why one good method of tapering down involves postponing the first cigarette of the day, which is the only one that doesn't have the additional "urge input" caused by a preceding cigarette.

One last word about nicotine addiction: here again many smokers look for a rationalization to allow themselves to continue to smoke. Many argue that since smoking is an addiction, they could never hope to lick it. Nonsense! Commit to the strategy you are reading and you will break your addiction in short order.

17. What should you know about "urges"?

Aside from enduring the discomforts of "withdrawal symptoms," the biggest fear of smokers thinking of stopping is that they won't be able to overcome tremendous desires, cravings and urges for a cigarette. Every smoker has already at least once had the experience of wanting desperately to smoke without being able to and knows how upsetting this can be. "Urges" to smoke might have appeared uncontrollable, coming out of nowhere, and intense enough to knock you over. Still, you *do* have immense control over these urges: their intensity, duration, frequency and eventual disappearance. As mentioned previously, you can also use taste signals (such as sucking candies) and olfactory signals to help you cope with these urges.

Much of what follows is aimed at the "urge" problem and how you can master it. Keep in mind that by "urge," I mean nothing more than an intense craving or desire to smoke. What is said applies no matter how you experience the craving (mildly, intensely, physically, etc.).

18. In quitting smoking, what should your goal be?

If you want to stop smoking, you should have in mind only one goal, and that is to reach a point fairly soon where smoking is no longer an issue for you, when urges to smoke disappear, when the chain of needing to smoke is off your neck completely, so that you are equivalent to a non-smoker. I don't feel that it makes sense to go into the task of quitting if you just see it as an endless, directionless adaptation of learning how to handle urge after urge for the rest of your life. Few people can sustain an effort like stopping smoking if it drags on very long. The initial commitment, energy, excitement, and resolve wear thin after a while, so the problem had better be finished quickly.

Even more important, it is very useful in doing anything to have a final goal, an endpoint to work toward. If stopping smoking seems endless and vague at the beginning, it is very hard to stick with it. You should set your sights on a goal – the goal of not having any urges – to see that you are working toward something that you value.

19. Can you count on being able to eliminate your cigarette cravings?

Absolutely. If you go about it the right way, you can be certain that within just one month of stopping, you will no longer have any urges.[‡] Actually, this one-month estimate is even high for most people. Many smokers stop having urges much sooner, but we will speak of one month because this will cover everybody.

I know that I am taking an extreme position in claiming you can stop having urges to smoke after so short a period, but I am convinced of this and will explain later why some people (who made some unfortunate errors while stopping) continue to experience strong desires to smoke two months or even two years after stopping (in Section 25).

Notice the relationship between what is being said here and many smokers' hopes

---

[‡] Later, I will refine and explain this a bit more carefully, but any modifications made will be extremely minor. Read on.

for magic. The magic many smokers hope for is that they will wake up one morning and no longer want to smoke. As discussed earlier, it isn't too wise to keep waiting for this. On the other hand, it seems to me pretty hopeful to think you can earn this result for yourself within so short a period of time – and without, by the way, the bouts of willpower you might think necessary.

20. Doesn't it make a difference how long or how much you've smoked?

No. Oddly enough, some of the people who have the easiest time quitting are two-pack-a-day 40-year smokers. Whether you inhale or not, whether your cigarette is strong or weak, whether filtered or not, and whatever your sex, age, education, or income, you can quit smoking and you can end your urges within a month.

21. How is it that you now "need" cigarettes?

Clearly, you weren't born with a "smoking drive." Moreover, your original reasons for starting smoking (usually social conformity, maturity, or independence were important back then) probably no longer operate. How is it, then, that you have come to have a craving for cigarettes perhaps every bit as strong as your inborn cravings for food and water? Apparently, something about your smoking behavior itself makes it self-sustaining.

There is the nicotine addiction and the psychological habit. From the psychological perspective you have a "need" for cigarettes because you've learned to have this need. A brief lesson in psychology will clarify this. You started out smoking only occasionally and probably didn't really enjoy it in the beginning. Beer, cigarettes, and coffee are all things that most of us originally forced ourselves to take for reasons other than enjoying them. By the hundredth cigarette, though, smoking was pleasant enough; and well before then you already would have trouble stopping. This is because you gradually, but repeatedly, paired cigarettes with all sorts of activities and emotions in your life combined with the hunger your body has developed for a nicotine fix.

It is by repeated pairings or associations that we learn. By always having a cigarette with a cup of coffee, or with a drink, or every telephone call; by never getting anxious, depressed or angry without taking a cigarette, you "learn" that cigarettes go with all of these activities and emotions. Some people almost always have a cup of coffee with a cigarette year after year. You can imagine how strong a link they have formed between coffee and cigarettes. Again, combine the habit with the power of nicotine to create a hunger in the body and the result is a strong desire to smoke.

When such people try to have a cup of coffee without a cigarette, it is understandable that they feel something is drastically wrong, something is missing –

and they can experience an intense craving for a cigarette. It is by the *repetition* of pairings between cigarettes and parts of your life along with the body hunger that you learn to "need" cigarettes. This kind of need is called an acquired drive and can be every bit as strong as a need you were born with, such as thirst.

22. What can we say about ending the "need"?

The goal that was mentioned earlier was to arrive at a point where you no longer have any cravings for cigarettes. This is the same thing as ending the "need" or "drive" for cigarettes. From what was said above, you can see that this amounts to undoing the links between cigarettes and the rest of your life.

We can take a lesson about how to accomplish this by looking back to how the cigarette need was originally learned: by gradual repeated pairings of cigarettes and their addictive nicotine content with your life's activities and emotions. To learn not to need cigarettes is to once again learn to pair "no-cigarette" with coffee, drinks, phone calls, waking up, anger, anxiety, and so on. This unpairing, therefore, begins when you stop smoking. Like when you first learned to smoke, you go successively from doing the activity even though it's uncomfortable and you must force yourself, to finding it okay, to feeling actually more comfortable with the new pattern.

By the mere repetition, now, of coffee with no-cigarette, you come to gradually break the coffee-cigarette link. Your first five coffees without a cigarette seem awful, almost unbearable; but by the fifteenth, it tastes just fine and you feel no craving. In other words, you *earn* the right to enjoy the fifteenth coffee without a cigarette exactly by putting up with the first (unpleasant) fourteen.

Many smokers have the impression that their smoking actually helps them enjoy things like drinks or coffees more than non-smokers do. If you are one of these people, you've played a sad trick on yourself. Like the heroin addict who needs heroin just to make life okay (and not better), you have learned to need a cigarette with a drink to enjoy it only as much as a non-smoker enjoys a drink alone. In the process of undoing the cigarette-drink pairing, you start out drastically interfering with your ability to enjoy the drink by not smoking, but end up by restoring the pleasure fully back to its original level, now without needing a cigarette. When you are a smoker, you don't heighten your pleasures beyond their natural levels – you become dependent on a cigarette just to keep them there. By enduring only a dozen or so repetitions of these pleasure experiences below their natural level because of not smoking, you gradually free yourself to return to that normal level without cigarettes.

23. Why doesn't it take as long to unlearn a habit as it does to learn it?

Some people wonder why it doesn't take ten years to break their smoking drive if they've been developing it for ten years. The answer lies in the fact that the original habit (smoking) didn't take ten years to be formed. Many of the thousands of repetitions did not go into strengthening the link – they were just supplementary.

Look at it this way: you spent your first fifteen or more years of life as a non-smoker. Your habit was non-smoking. Yet, it didn't take fifteen years to undo that habit and replace it with the new one of smoking. All that is necessary to replace one habit with another is to be willing to disrupt things for a month or so and enforce a new, unnatural pattern on yourself for that time. Then it, just by virtue of repeating the new pattern, will become your new *natural* pattern.

24. How does the unlearning work?

Remember that we have discussed the fact that your only reasonable goal is to work toward making urges stop happening soon. How do you get rid of a recurring urge? To answer this, it will be helpful to return again to some psychological understanding that has dealt with other urges besides smoking.

A great deal of attention has been paid to a consistent, but surprising, war phenomenon. It is very common that soldiers who were lost during battle for, say, a week have lost their hunger drive. When found, these men literally had to be reminded to eat. The psychological understanding of this is clearly useful for us, in wanting to find a way to lose a smoking drive. This understanding can be briefly stated: if you ignore any urge long enough, it will go away.

The word "ignore" is very important. The soldier lost in battle is not eating; but on top of that, he's not thinking about eating because he is constantly thinking about something else – whether he will be captured or rescued, whether he will survive. This constant obsession forces out of his mind his concern for his stomach. It takes but a couple of days of ignoring the hunger

urge (not eating and not thinking about it) to
make it wither away.

The same thing is true, by the way, of
political prisoners on hunger strikes and
even Gandhi doing his forty-day fast. They
all report, as you may know, that within a
couple of days they experience no hunger at
all. Here also are the same ingredients: not
eating and not thinking about it because of
constant attention to other issues (in this
case, political ideals).

The same thing is true of some smokers.
Those people you know of who one day
threw away their cigarettes and didn't suffer
at all had this experience precisely because
their decision to quit was firm enough not to
allow themselves opportunities later to re-
negotiate their decision or let themselves
dwell on it. This was discussed in Section
5e. These people differ from those who have
great difficulties in stopping only in terms of
how much they let themselves think about
smoking once they've quit. The difference
between them is *not* in willpower (I'm sure
you know many smokers who want to stop

who don't impress you as having such
strong willpower). As you'll see below,
willpower need not and should not play a
role in stopping smoking.

25. How important is "not thinking about it"?

This element is crucial. Let me prove it.

Imagine now another soldier, also lost at
battle, but this time, with one apple with him
when lost. Imagine that he cuts up the apple
in many small pieces and rations them out to
himself over the course of a week. Notice
how this is like tapering down: he waits for
the food, anticipates it, constantly thinks
about it, and finds it very rewarding when he
has each bit. At the end of a week, as you
will agree, this soldier will be *starving*. One
soldier is not hungry and the other is
starving at the end of the week. What
accounts for this difference? Certainly it's
not the difference in how much they ate (one
little apple for a whole week!). The
difference lies in how much each thought

about eating: one not at all and the other all the time.

This difference is also important in understanding those ex-smokers you know who continue to have strong urges to smoke months or years after they stop. I have spoken to many of them and have invariably found that even though they have not smoked, they readily discuss those many times when they sit imagining themselves smoking, stand near smokers to breathe in their smoke, imagine themselves making smoke rings, and so on. These unfortunate people (who deserve a lot of credit for maintaining their energy not to give in for such a long period of time) are unwittingly prolonging their struggle by these seemingly innocent fantasies.

By the way, there's another reason not to be discouraged by these people's difficulties. They are undoubtedly reporting to you experiences of cravings maybe only once every few weeks – not the forty-a-day you may fear having when you first stop.

Actually, I think you would agree on the importance of not thinking about smoking once you stop, even without referring to these examples. If you would have fifteen cups of coffee while only just imagining you were smoking, it's clear that you would keep the coffee-smoking link alive and still desire a cigarette with the next cup.

26. Does this mean you now have two jobs to do?

When you originally thought about stopping, you may have thought this amounted just to not smoking anymore, forever enduring the same thing, just maybe somehow getting used to it. I've already shown you that quitting is not this endless, goalless task, and that there is a reasonable and attainable goal to work toward (having no more urges). What is also being said is that you must do two jobs to achieve this: not smoke and not think about it. Certainly you are asking *how* not to think about it – and this will be covered later.

For now it is useful to point out that the new task of "not thinking about it" really doesn't increase your work, because not thinking about it actually makes it trivially easy not to smoke.

27. How can you make an urge go away?

By not thinking about it! Happily, the same technique that makes urges stop occurring eventually will also make each and every current urge go away. If you can turn your attention off an urge, that urge is gone. You've probably already experienced this. Most people who have ever tried to curtail their smoking have gone through an unbearably long period of craving a cigarette – maybe an hour or more. And then they've also discovered, much to their surprise, that another couple of hours have gone by without their even noticing that they haven't smoked. This was usually because they "got too busy with something else." What we want to do is capitalize on this kind of situation and *make* it happen instead of waiting for it to happen.

You see, there are three things you can do with any urge:

- You can give in to it (smoke),
- you can fight it,
- you can ignore it.

Unfortunately, most would-be-quitters have gone the "fight it" route. This involves that familiar sweat-and-blood, battle-to-the-death, lengthy and painful struggle of pitting the two sides of yourself against each other. "I don't want to smoke…yes, I do…oh, I'm dying for a cigarette…maybe just one…no, it's not the thing to do…but one wouldn't matter…well, try to wait a few more minutes…oh, but I really do want a cigarette…" etc., etc. These kinds of battles can last well up to several hours and are incredibly painful. This is where willpower plays a role: you must exercise sheer brute force of will not to give in during such a painful battle.

What is crucial to realize is that 1) these battles (and, therefore, willpower) are completely unnecessary and, moreover 2) they are harmful to your efforts. They are *harmful* because even though negative thoughts, you are still thinking about cigarettes through the whole battle. Even if you don't fantasize *positive* images of smoking, you can still keep your urges coming forever because of these battleground experiences of thinking about smoking – and even if you win them all and continue not to smoke! The willpower quitter deserves a medal for withstanding all the torture, but he unwittingly prolongs his cravings well beyond the month we've been referring to – and this, merely because he battled those urges.

It is not necessary to battle urges. If you ignore them – stop thinking about them – they will fade (again, how to do this will be discussed soon). Many smokers conceive of their recurrent feelings of craving as repeated emergences of brewing inside and that each time they manage to postpone smoking, they are just increasing the tension and pressure inside and that the craving will just grow and grow until it will eventually get them. This is nonsense. If you ignore an urge at 3:00 and it goes away and if you again get an urge at 4:00, this is a new and different urge.

Think about it. There's no cubbyhole inside your head where one urge is sitting, waiting to come out again and again. Each time you get an urge to smoke, this is a new urge. What is an urge anyhow? It's nothing more than an awareness that you are not smoking and want to. As soon as that awareness is gone, the urge is gone; as soon as you are no longer thinking about wanting to smoke, you don't *want* to smoke anymore.

An urge stays with you exactly as long as you choose to attend to it. Yes, people have two-hour-long urges. They realize that they want to smoke and just sit there and have an incredible battle about it. The *instant* they take their mind off that arena, the urge is gone. Another urge may come later (or even very soon), but this is a different urge and it too will disappear as soon as you are able to stop thinking about it.

Let me say this all one more way. A craving for a cigarette when trying to stop or cut down can be almost unbearable. You can feel almost like it's going to knock you over, like you're practically going to drop dead if you don't have a cigarette soon. It is perfectly reasonable to want desperately to terminate this feeling. I would never urge anyone just to bear up and be strong enough to live through such cravings. They can be murder. But there are *two* ways to make an urge go away: by smoking or by not smoking! We usually tell ourselves that we *must* take a cigarette to make the dread craving go away. This is not so. You *should* want to make the urge go away, but you don't have to do that by taking a cigarette. If you *ignore* the urge, it will also go away.

To summarize, "the right way" to stop smoking, both for the short-term (to make an urge go away) and for the long-term (to make urges stop coming), is to *ignore* every urge. How do you do that?

28. How can you ignore urges?

You cannot not-think about something by deciding not to think about it. If you decide not to think about your nose for the next three seconds, that's exactly what you *will* think about. Still, there is a way to control what you think about and this comes from the fact that it is impossible to attend simultaneously to two different thoughts (although we do sometimes quickly alternate between two thoughts). To not think about smoking, you must think about something else.

You should take this idea seriously and make a practiced technique out of it. Make a list for yourself (perhaps not necessarily written) of fantasies, puzzles, observations, issues that are interesting for you. Have some ideas prepared so that the second you get an urge to smoke, you can rush into one of these other thoughts. Be ready, every time you get an urge, to quickly (and artificially) direct your focus to a different arena. Imagine what it would be like to be Queen of England, or to be in the Foreign Legion. Think about what you could buy if you had to spend one million dollars in 24 hours. Muse about where you would like to go for a "dream" vacation, how you would change your appearance if you could, etc. Ask yourself how many days there are between January 12th and March 15th. Try to remember the states in alphabetical order. Pay attention to the noises you are hearing wherever you are, or the smells. Count the stitches somewhere in your clothing, or the dots on the ceiling, or whatever.

Take this seriously. This is a specific technique I'm suggesting – and it works. You need not have a rich or colorful fantasy life, nor dream in Technicolor, for it to work for you. And you can do it anywhere, under any circumstances. When first hearing of this procedure, many people have objected that they have a busy day at work and don't have time to sit daydreaming about the

Sahara Desert. What they don't realize is that this takes no time at all. The very instant you turn your attention on to the competing thought, your urge is gone and you can return to your usual business. The second you "hook" onto the other thought, your craving has been broken. One man reported to me that every time he got an urge for a whole week, he started planning a vacation – and at the end of the week, he still hadn't picked the country, because each time he never had to stay with it long enough.

The suggestion I am making is not just a vague "Every time you feel like smoking, think about something else." It's a well-defined and powerful technique you must take seriously and practice. Really have a list of thoughts prepared in advance. One woman worked out a very mechanical technique. She wrote down, in her appointment book, a list of twelve thoughts and numbered them 2 through 13. Each time she got an urge to smoke, she reached for the book, looked over the page, and chose an item, saying, for example, "This time it's

Number 8" and off she went in a new
thought. Whether you choose such a
rigorous version or not, you should see it as
a careful and planned procedure.

The process should be: getting in touch
with the craving for a cigarette and then
immediately turning on another thought.
Don't include a middle ground of urge-
battling or reminding yourself, "Oh yes, I'm
not supposed to think about smoking; that
book said not to; it's bad for me to think
about a cigarette, etc.," because all this still
involves thinking about smoking. You
literally should be able to go to bed at night
knowing that you didn't think about
smoking at all the whole day for more than a
few seconds, or minutes.

The alternate thoughts you choose
should have three characteristics. One, they
should be compelling for you, able to attract
your attention. One person can get involved
in thinking about being an operatic star, but
this would leave someone else cold. Second,
the thought should not in itself set off an
urge for a cigarette. Some would do well

fantasizing about getting a million dollars, but others – who have paired smoking with handling money problems – would feel an urge because of this thought. Finally, and obvious enough, your thought should not include cigarettes or smoking in the content. Don't count matches, count pretzels.

29. Will this work for you?

Right this moment, you can't yet be sure. But be assured that this alternate-focus procedure does work. You won't be able to feel the sense of mastery it gives until maybe you've gone through seven times when you yourself see that you can make an urge go away as soon as you want to. As you can imagine, you will then have a great sense of comfort about the ease of handling urges.

True, you do not have control over when urges will occur and how strong they will be. Urges are ignited for a variety of reasons. You may get physical sensations (such as those involved in "coming down" from an earlier cigarette-induced rush of nicotine hunger). You may feel an urge from seeing other people smoke or even just a pack of cigarettes. You may feel an emotion which you had tied to smoking and this can set off an urge. You may do an activity (drink coffee, talk on the phone) and kindle an urge.

Wherever the urge came from, no matter how strong it is, and no matter how soon it comes following an urge just before it, you can kill the urge the same way – by not thinking about it! You don't have control about the onset of an urge, but you can terminate every single one of them at will! The procedure, I might add, is extremely easy to do, and it works; but so is smoking a cigarette easy and efficient in ending an urge. The choice is up to you: you now have two easy ways to end urges. The difference between remaining a smoker and becoming an ex-smoker (who comes quickly to resemble a non-smoker) lies in the choice that you make.

Let me finish this section with a personal example. One day, after not smoking for only a couple of weeks, I got a very upsetting telephone call. There was a pack of cigarettes sitting on a table across the room from me. I don't know if it was because I had a triple input making up this urge (telephone call link, upset, and visibility of cigarettes), but it felt like about the strongest urge I had experienced. I told myself, really, that I would just about drop dead if I didn't have a cigarette, and fast! Forget the stopping smoking, forget the two weeks off, forget the Surgeon General – I *needed* a cigarette. And so I started across the room, trying to stretch enough so I could grab the pack without letting go of the phone (I'm sure you know the scene well). Luckily, I remembered halfway across the room that there was an alternate, but equally efficient, way to end my agony. Since I couldn't really get myself to fantasize about being King of Spain at that moment, I tried just listening for an instant to the tone of voice of the person on the phone, instead of the content of what was being said, which was so upsetting. I just listened for highs and lows, and volume. Well, two seconds later, I was still in the same room, with the same bad news, talking with the same person on the same phone, and the same pack of cigarettes was sitting in the same place. But the idea of smoking left me completely cold. Nothing had changed, but I broke the craving.

I know from my own experience and from the experience of hundreds of people I've worked with: this technique works. When people now tell me that they *had* to smoke a certain cigarette, I can sympathize with the pain, but I also know they had a potent alternative to smoking to make the pain stop.

30. How often will you have urges when you first stop?

While frequency of urges varies greatly from person to person, a general pattern does show up. Many people report that on the first days off cigarettes, they have to deal with a fairly constant awareness that they are not smoking – a constant hovering awareness that something is wrong, something is missing. Like withdrawal symptoms, this unavoidable unpleasantness just simply must be endured. It is manageable because of the awareness and certainty that it will be very temporary. By the second, or certainly third, day there is already a great improvement. Urges may come very frequently, but you start to notice that major time periods go by where you haven't at all thought about smoking. Urges come and go, although they may be as frequent as 40 or 50 times a day. But now they are manageable – because you can turn them off as soon as you turn to something else.

A few days later, you will have maybe only half as many urges a day. By the end of the first week, there will probably be only 10-20 urges a day. After two weeks, it will probably be less than five; by three weeks, only one or two a day and then only one every couple of days. And then, if you haven't smoked *at all* in a month, and if you haven't let yourself think about smoking (either positively or negatively), you will have *no more urges.*

This is a general pattern; for many people, the decline goes much faster. For a few people, the peak may not be the first day. They may experience more and more urges through the first three or four days before they peak and begin their decline. If your third day is worse than the first, don't be scared or discouraged. It will not continue to grow this way. You too will soon begin to see urges decrease day by day.

31. How intense will the urges be?

When you first stop smoking, you will definitely notice that urges come less and less frequently. Unfortunately, the intensity of urges does not follow the same curve as does the frequency of urges. This means that an urge you experience after two weeks may feel just as strong as one you felt the second day. Don't let this throw you, because the technique you have for handling urges works *no matter* how intense an urge may be. The greatest danger coming from the fact that urges don't decrease in intensity during the first month is that this is often used as a rationalization for going back. People say that there has been no progress because urges feel as strong as ever, sometimes as if they could knock you over. Look at the frequency of these urges to reassure yourself that tremendous progress has seen made.

32. Can you take an occasional cigarette when you first stop?

Absolutely not. If you accept all the above reasoning about breaking your cigarette links and how it is done, you must also accept one important implication: "Cheating" will strongly disrupt the process.

Once again, your goal is to become equivalent to a non-smoker, to no longer have any urges. There is only one way to do this: not smoke and not think about smoking until the links are broken (one month or less). This means you have a bout of work to do for one solid month, using an efficient technique that removes the task away from the arena of battling urges by using brute willpower.

If you were to take just one cigarette during the month, you would pay heavily for it. First of all, it would be tremendously difficult to make it be just *one* cigarette (more about this later). More important, you would be lengthening the time period when you will continue to have urges.

Suppose you are someone who will have to wait the full four weeks before the urges stop (this varies from person to person and also depends on how good you are at not thinking about cigarettes). If you were to take one cigarette two weeks into the period, you would rekindle a lot of the link strength you had been undoing. Certainly you wouldn't undo the whole two weeks' progress, but you may well insure that you have a whole extra weeks worth of urges to handle. It's impossible to prove this, because it's impossible to measure these things. Still, I'm convinced that one cigarette along the way may make you a five-week person, instead of a four-week person. A whole week's worth of urges just from one cigarette! Indeed, you could keep urges alive for the rest of your life by smoking just one pack a year, one cigarette every couple of weeks. By pushing yourself just a couple of more weeks, though, you could be finished with cravings forever.

There is another, rather complicated reason why taking an occasional cigarette when you first stop can cost you plenty. It will require a mini-psychology lesson to explain.

Let us turn for a moment to a psychology animal laboratory. It is common to do research on learning by using rats in cages. It is easy to train a rat to regularly press a bar in his cage by reinforcing this act with a drop of water, assuming the animal is thirsty. Sometimes, the rat is given water *every* time he presses the bar. This is called *continuous* reinforcement. Another possibility is to give water only after several bar-presses. Thus, the rat presses the bar once, twice, three times and gets no water; but maybe the fourth will yield his reward. It turns out that animals trained this way (called *intermittent* reinforcement) press the bar much more frequently!

A more striking difference between these two methods of reinforcement comes later. After training both ways, researchers study the effect of turning off the water altogether. An animal trained with continuous reinforcement will keep pressing the bar for a while even with no more water; then he will stop. One given intermittent reinforcement will also stop pressing eventually after the water is turned off, but much, much later. It is impressive to watch these latter animals press the bar maybe hundreds of times without any more reward forthcoming. The name for the process of what happens after turning off the reward is "extinction." The scientific way of saying what was just explained is that "intermittent reinforcement is much more resistant to extinction than is continuous reinforcement."

If you now think of an *urge* as a *bar-press* and *taking a cigarette* as the *reinforcement*, you will see what this means. If you train yourself to intermittently reinforce urges with cigarettes, you will both increase the frequency of urges and guarantee that urges will continue to occur for a long time after you finally fully turn off the cigarette supply. Once again, you pay very heavily for taking occasional cigarettes.

Back in the beginning of this article, it was mentioned that a strong commitment to whatever goal you choose will make your job easier. Let us apply that now. Commit yourself to not smoking or thinking about it for one solid month. Really plan to stick to this, *no matter what!* If you ever plan to stop smoking, you will have to log up on a solid month like this, and if you go into it with intense resolve to last the whole month, you will get the additional ease that comes with firm non-changeable commitment.

33. What occurs in the process of stopping?

You will be able to watch three things changing in the course of your initial month off cigarettes.

First, as discussed earlier, the frequency of urges will change drastically from many a day in the beginning to none at all at the end. This is repeated here because the occurrence of urges to smoke can be used as another rationalization for going back. You will almost certainly have urges to smoke up until the end of the month. Don't tell yourself that things aren't going right if you still have urges after two weeks. This is normal. Remember that it is your final goal not to have urges anymore and that by not smoking you are working towards this goal. It doesn't happen along the way.

Similarly, don't tell yourself things aren't working just because you miss cigarettes in your life. Yes, coffees or drinks may not be enjoyable in the beginning. In the beginning you may feel a big void in your life, like something is terribly missing. Don't let *this* feeling send you back to smoking, because your reaction to not smoking is the second thing that changes in the first month. In the beginning, coffee is awful without cigarettes; in the end, it tastes just fine. It is by enduring the unpleasantness that you reach your goal of comfort at the end of the month.

Finally, your reaction to the thought of never smoking again changes during the month. This whole issue will be discussed later, but an important point must be made now. If you feel panic at the thought of never smoking again, this is reasonable enough. You still have urges to smoke and the thought of never smoking again may indeed feel terrifying. Don't let this *feeling* interfere with your work, because the feeling will change. At the *end* of the month, when you have no more urges, you will no longer feel terrified about never smoking again. In fact, you're likely to feel delighted. You will be a different person after quitting for a month, experiencing no more urges. You will care as much then about not being able to smoke as you care now about not being able to experiment with heroin. Once again, you must guard against that familiar illogic: "I can maybe go without smoking for a month, but one day or another I'll give in to this panic about *never* smoking again, so I might as well do it now." The panic feeling will not always be there – it is just another reflection of still having urges to smoke.

34. When should you stop?

The stage is now set for you. You know what is involved in stopping, you know what your goal is, you know how to achieve it, and you know how to understand and minimize your suffering. All that remains is deciding when to stop. As you know, this is an important issue.

If you were asked whether you want to be a non-smoker a year from now, you would certainly answer "yes." That's an easy one. What you must acknowledge to yourself now is that for this to happen, you must do your month's bout of work somewhere between now and a year from now. Smokers can let years at a time go by, waiting for their non-smoking to just happen to them before accepting that it just won't happen. You will not be a non-smoker a year from now if you just wait for it to happen; if you just wait for a day when the plunge won't seem so big. As mentioned earlier, even the jump from five cigarettes a day to none is a big plunge that you must consciously undertake; stopping requires an active decision – you don't just slip into it.

So now, when should you plunge into your "getting off" month? Any date you choose will have its advantages and disadvantages. No month you set aside will be perfectly conflict-free. In a sense, no date is better than any other date.

Let me report my own experience in deciding when to stop – it will probably sound familiar. At midnight, say, on August 5th, I would say to myself that this is it! Now is when I stop smoking. I would throw away all my cigarettes, clean all the ashtrays and put them away, and make many announcements of my plans to my friends.

Then comes the next morning. After coffee and breakfast, I start to have a tremendous desire for a cigarette (naturally). So I ask myself what was so special about the moment, August 5th at midnight? Why don't I have just one more cigarette (as if this were going to be the last craving of my life) and then do my quitting at 10 a.m. on August 6th? The only end to this game came when I realized that I would always fail in looking for some reason, some justification, for choosing any one moment to stop. There is no God-given magic moment to stop smoking. If you wait for one, or try to find a special reason for any particular moment you choose, you'll be lost.

Still, you must choose a time – and stick with it. Everyone who has successfully stopped smoking has actually done something that on the surface looks irrational. It is difficult to explain why it's alright to smoke as much as you want before the "quit" moment and then no more afterwards. Don't look for explanations, but like all quitters, choose a moment and then put all your energy into that moment.

It is critical that you not allow yourself to abandon the moment you originally select. It is true that you will probably be able to find some very good reason for moving your quit time to some later new time. People pick a moment to stop and then tell themselves that they should reconsider and start to stop later because: they just had a fight with their boss, they are having their house painted, the kids are especially loud today, and so on. People decide they mustn't try to stop on a work day because of the pressures of the job. Then, on the chosen Friday night, they reason they shouldn't spoil their weekend with quitting because it's the only peace they have all week, and so on. They decide that out-of-town guests, cigarettes remaining in a package, or a wedding celebration are all good causes for postponing quitting. It's endless. If you find a good reason to abandon a moment you've chosen in favor of a second moment, you'll certainly be able to find another reason, just as good, to abandon the new choice.

Indeed, a good rule of thumb is to ask yourself, when contemplating a postponement because of a certain reason, "Won't I be able to think of an even better reason for another postponement later?" Practically by definition, you have continued to smoke exactly because you've allowed yourself to endlessly postpone the moment of quitting.

Let's get concrete. As of this very moment, make a decision, a very firm decision. Choose a day within the next seven days (you don't need longer; if you're thinking you do, it's almost certainly because you're continuing the postponement pattern) when you will quit. Don't let anything move you off of your choice. In preparation for that day, you have three possible choices: 1) smoke as usual, then stop at the chosen moment, 2) taper down in preparation for that day – and the tapering down method discussed in Section 9 is recommended, or 3) smoke considerably more than usual until the chosen time, so that in a sense (but only for the very beginning period of quitting) you'll feel relieved not to smoke.

Remember, once again: it is crucial that you stick to the time that you've selected. One postponement will open the door to many, many others.

Good luck.

35. Suggested Reading Instructions

It is recommended that you stop reading this book now, before going on to the next section on staying off. Decide when you're going to quit (within the next seven days). Then, just before that moment, you may want to go back and re-read the portions of the section on getting off that are likely to encourage you or guide you.

Then, after you haven't smoked for about a week, go on to read the rest of the book.

III. STAYING OFF

As you know, a high proportion of those who stop smoking go back again. Does this mean that they stopped the wrong way at first? No. Stopping and staying off are two separate processes and no method of stopping will in itself guarantee maintenance. Maintenance must be given its own attention. Many people go back to smoking for one plain reason: it is very easy to go back. Luckily, it is also *very* easy not to go back, once cravings have disappeared.

36. How is staying off different from getting off?

As discussed earlier, the beginning period of stopping smoking may involve withdrawal symptoms, intense cravings, and a major commitment to stick with it. This is a period of intensity. There are strong pushes and pulls on you in all sorts of directions. Then, within a month or less, the cravings stop, the symptoms stop, and it is rare that you even focus your attention on smoking. Your life feels as full without cigarettes as it previously felt only with the help of regular smoking. The thought of not smoking anymore delights you, instead of sending chills of panic through your spine.

In this period of getting off, those who don't make it and go back again do so because they feel the need to eliminate some pain (craving, symptoms, etc.). They give in to the pulling –yanking around – they feel from the intensity of their desire to smoke and not to smoke.

After the getting-off period, the situation is very different. It then becomes a simple matter of making a decision – a calm decision. The decision about whether to smoke a cigarette is really very mild: the idea of smoking is just that – an idea. It is not backed up by any violent, earth-shattering craving. Nearly everyone who goes back to smoking after a month or more off reports the same thing. They thought about smoking just one cigarette and decided that it would cause no harm. They agree that it would have caused no pain or hardship to pass it up, but really couldn't see any harm in it. There is a lot of harm, as we'll see below, but notice how different the situation is.

When you first get off cigarettes, you may blow it because you give in to strong pulls on you to smoke. To go back later involves only making the wrong decision, because of not having enough information to make a sound decision.

37. What information should you have to guarantee staying off?

You must know (and believe) that it is not "safe" to smoke "just one cigarette." Ex-smokers have come up with a thousand reasonable-sounding arguments about why they can smoke a cigarette once they've been off for a while:

"I've licked it, I'm not having any more urges, I'm safe now, so there's no harm taking just one cigarette."

"I owe it to myself to see what a cigarette would taste like now, just as a scientific experiment so to speak."

"I've done so well, not smoking for so long – I owe myself a little reward; I'll just take one cigarette."

"I've proven I can control myself now so it's certain I'll be able to smoke just one cigarette without it getting out of control."

Practically no one smokes just one cigarette more after stopping. For most, that one cigarette becomes the royal road to inching back up to normal smoking patterns, more or less slowly. Some others (unfortunately a small minority) observe how quickly they start re-escalating their smoking and quickly make a new decision to stop again. They are amazed and disappointed to see that the second quitting (even if it's when they're only back up to a couple of cigarettes a day) is full-fledged quitting, often as hard as the first one. It may even be harder because they don't have nearly as much energy to bring to the task

and find it hard to get too excited over a
two-or-three-a-day habit.

38. Why isn't it "just one cigarette"?

It is pretty easy to understand why
smoking "just one cigarette" is so nearly
impossible.

a. There is certain "staying power" in the
accomplishment of many smoke-less days.
When you're off three, or six, or ten weeks,
your pride buoys you on to continue. Should
something come up (an urge, a rationalization)
that is potent enough to get you to smoke
despite this "staying power," it will also be
potent enough to let you smoke a second
cigarette 30 minutes later. To put it another
way, once you break a six-week fast, it's
nothing to break a 30-minute fast, 30 minutes
later, when you will probably experience an
urge. And don't forget, the nicotine in those
cigarettes is itching to get hold of you, and it is
likely that it will.

b. Even though you may have stopped
having urges, one smoke is enough to

rekindle them. This is partially physical and was already discussed before and as you are being reminded above. Your physical "coming down" from the adrenalin flow of your first "cheat" may well signal a craving half an hour later. More generally, urges do wither away if you give them long enough, but can easily be reignited (by smoking). Remember those soldiers lost at war who lost their hunger drive. Had they continued not to eat once rescued, they still would not have experienced hunger pangs – and would even die of starvation. But give them just one meal and their hunger drive will begin to return. After a couple of days of normal eating, they'll be hungry as often as the rest of us. It's the same with cigarettes.

   c. Most people report unpleasant sensations when they first take a cigarette after a period of abstinence. They say it tastes awful, makes their heart pound, and makes them dizzy. (As an aside, let me point out here that all cigarettes do this to all smokers, but a regular smoker is so deadened to such sensations that he doesn't experience these same physical upheavals.) (As another aside, let me mention one man I heard of whose death was caused by "just one cigarette." His first cigarette after a few weeks off was while driving. It overwhelmed him so that he fainted – and crashed.)

In terms of psychological learning theory, one might assume that such an unpleasant result of smoking one's first "cheat" as extreme dizziness might turn one off to ever smoking again. Unfortunately, it seems that other, somewhat amusing, forces are usually more powerful. The disappointed "cheater" says to himself, "I hate myself, I feel miserable, I blew it, I smoked a cigarette and now feel all these guilty feelings. And I didn't even enjoy it. I'll be darned if I'm going to bear such guilt for something I didn't even enjoy. I'm going to at least smoke another one that I'll enjoy to make my bad feelings fit the sin." Before he knows it, he's into his third or fourth cigarette.

d. Many people initially experience what they feel is success with "just one cigarette." They manage to take one and no more for a few days. Taking this as proof of their ability to smoke "just one cigarette," then they smoke another "just one cigarette" (not bothering to count that this is their second cigarette). Again they experience what they feel is success and begin to feel that they will be able to smoke every so often like this. Already they've gone from the "just one cigarette" myth to the "occasional cigarette" myth. One night, when out drinking, they smoke several cigarettes and since they manage not to smoke the next day, they begin to decide they're going to be able to smoke freely while drinking without it getting out of control in other circumstances. Now they're adopting the "occasional cigarette and occasion-tied smoking" myth. As you can see, it isn't long before they've added free smoking after meals, when upset, on vacation with smoking friends, at card games, etc. – oops – before they know it they're at a pack a day.

So, a successful "just one cigarette" smoker isn't successful at all. His "success" lures him to failure, and this can be more or less slowly.

39. Why can't you become an occasional smoker now?

We've covered this already somewhat in Section 8. Now let's look again at the question from the point of view of someone who hasn't smoked for a month or more and has broken his links. It is tempting to reason that the slate is clean and you can start up a new smoking habit at whatever (low) level you choose.

First of all, consider the fact that you began smoking like everyone else – very slowly; only a few cigarettes a day. Among the group of people who have at least once lit up a cigarette there are three subcategories which have formed: Group I – those who never touched another one; Group II – those who continue to smoke *ir*regularly and less than 5 or 10 a day and never smoke more; and Group III – those of us who went on to become regular, "hooked" smokers. Who knows why a given person goes one route or the other? There is talk about "addictive personalities," oral needs, and so on, and one day we may be able to answer this question.

For now, all you should ask yourself is this: if you didn't stop in Group 2 your first time around, why do you think you'll be able to now?

Psychological and physiological theories provide another explanation for your not being able to become an occasional smoker now. It is widely believed that there are *physical* neural brain connections formed corresponding to all of our learning. Smoking also stimulates "reward centers" of the brain providing a temporary addictive pleasure that carries a terrible long-term price. It doesn't seem far-fetched, therefore, to assume that we are all "wired" (by our own doing and experience) to be a certain kind of smoker.

This is backed up by the fact that most smokers who stop for a long period and return to smoking settle back in at the same rate per day. Notice also that smokers smoke roughly the same number of cigarettes on a weekend day, work day, or vacation day – even though their stresses and situations vary widely. It's a bit like learning to ride a bicycle. Even after 20 years, someone who gets on a bike will slip into riding it very easily. Maybe those neural connections are there and, if so, we can either stop them from firing (by staying off cigarettes, or the bicycle) or else the juice will all start flowing again and in the same way.

40. What if you do smoke a cigarette?

Does the above reasoning mean that taking "just one cigarette" is the same thing as going back to smoking? And that you might as well start up full-steam as soon as you do "cheat" once, because you'll get there sooner or later anyhow? Of course not.

If you *do* cheat (which is to be strongly discouraged), acknowledge it as such and then set your mind on *stopping* again. I use the words "stopping again" on purpose: you really should think of yourself as a smoker who must quit smoking even as soon as the first cigarette. This is because you indeed must muster up again pretty much all the energy that quitting requires because even just one cigarette will throw your way all sorts of forces aimed at becoming a regular smoker again and you have to have your own forces in gear to take them on.

If you should cheat once, you won't *automatically* be a regular smoker again but you will have unleashed significant tendencies to get there quickly and you'll have to be prepared to take them on. So in contemplating a "cheat," be fully aware that it will lead to one of two "heavy" or unpleasant consequences: a return to smoking regularly (thereby throwing away all your earlier work and difficulties) or another new major task that you'll have to face.

41. Will you really never have another urge?

All along, as you have been reading, you have gotten the guarantee that if you log a month of not smoking and not thinking about it, you will have no more cravings to smoke – assuming there are no "cheats." To a very small extent, this was a misrepresentation, and you should know the whole story now. For the entire rest of your life, after this month's work, you will never again have another urge – except perhaps for five or so more times, total.

These few exceptions are understandable and it is important that you know about them so that they won't surprise you and you'll be able to handle them. The exceptions are those that may occur in peak, super-special difficult experiences. Many ex-smokers experience their first urge in months, for example, when involved in a car accident, major argument, airplane scare, or other stress occurrence. This really is not inconsistent with the explanation of how urges die out. Links are broken because of repetitions of life experiences without cigarettes, and not just the passage of time. Normally, in the month of undoing links (luckily), you won't have had a chance to undo your peak crisis-cigarette link. Still, if you would be put through five car crashes without smoking, you wouldn't crave a cigarette anymore in the sixth.

Naturally these particular cravings are especially difficult. While you are exchanging insurance information with the other driver, you won't much feel like imagining what it would be like to be the Queen of England. Still, you *must not smoke*. This is because all of the usual understanding and mechanisms involved with "just one cigarette" are still at work. You must force yourself, however difficult it may be, to remember that the intense craving will go away even if you don't smoke, once you are able to get your mind off it. Further, it will help to remember that this unusual craving is one of just a handful you'll have to handle for the whole rest of your life – unless you smoke, that is. On the other hand, if you do smoke, you won't have to wait long for the next urge to come.

There is one more thing you should know and remember – something many others have borne painful testimony to. If you do smoke in a crisis situation, in fact, you'll be much worse off than if you don't smoke. Taking a cigarette after a car accident will make the craving go away (for about ten minutes, maybe) but it won't make the accident go away. You'll still be in the same miserable situation, but worse! On top of the painful feeling related to the accident, you'll feel a surge of misery at the fact that you smoked. Earlier, we mentioned that the negative consequences of smoking don't come consistently or immediately enough. The crisis cigarette after being off for a long time will consistently and immediately cause you considerable pain. If you really know and accept this in advance, you'll be able to abstain even though the temptation may be great, especially when you consider that you can count the number of the exceptional remaining intense cravings on the fingers of one hand.

42. Is it impossible to go back to smoking after the cravings stop?

Of course not. Unfortunately, there will never be any invisible protective shield in front of your mouth blocking the passage to any and all cigarettes. Furthermore, you should expect that cigarettes will always be available throughout your lifetime. But don't be afraid. Once the urges stop, it's incredibly easy not to go back to smoking. It's just that it's also very easy to go back, too.

Let me speak here of my own experience. Every so often (usually at parties), I find myself saying to myself, "I bet I'd enjoy a cigarette right now." And I'm sure I would. But half-a-second behind that thought is the thought that I'm not going to smoke because I would pay too heavily for that cigarette. There is no panic, no sense of deprivation, no crisis. The thought is gone as fast and as painlessly as it came.

Compare this to other experiences of your own. I'm sure you have plenty of temptations, whether it be spending, cutting some legal corners or having an affair. And I'm sure the thought occurs to you to yield. But the thought that it's out of the question and that you would pay too heavily for this act doesn't come far behind. You, therefore, don't stop in your tracks, trying to decide what to do; no beads of perspiration form on your forehead as you contemplate your next move. Some of those temptations are stronger than grabbing a cigarette after you have successfully quit. If you manage those temptations, you can certainly manage not to reach for a cigarette.

Likewise, I assume you don't give much thought to, nor suffer from, not experimenting with heroin. You understand that the first few fixes are pretty enjoyable, but your knowledge of the consequences serves to make it incredibly easy not to look to heroin for enjoyment.

43. What distinguishes the people who relapse from those who stay off?

The line is drawn fairly clearly. Those people who get off of cigarettes and never go back again, in my experience, are always those who would agree that they cannot ever smoke again, even just one cigarette (or rather, *especially* "just one cigarette"). On the other side, those who do go back almost always are the people who don't quite accept this prohibition. Actually, there are a few others who go back consciously deciding to become a smoker again, but almost all relapses start out with a desire to remain a non-smoker, except for one cigarette.

The reports of the gradual return to smoking are fairly uniform and often humorous. "I just took one cigarette for the hell of it and then another one a few days later. I started bumming cigarettes every so often, secure in the knowledge that I wasn't really a smoker as long as I didn't buy any cigarettes. When I felt I was getting a little obnoxious with all my bumming, I would buy a pack for my friend – but of course they weren't really my cigarettes. Then, one day, no friends were around to buy for or bum from and so…"

In case you are reading these lines during a period when you are still smoking, or only recently quit, remember that the idea of never smoking again will *not* cause a panic reaction once your urges stop. Wait a month after stopping until you try to commit yourself to never smoking again. But then, you must come to accept this idea.

Perhaps it sounds overly harsh and conservative. Perhaps you could smoke only two or three more cigarettes the rest of your life (I doubt it). Is it worth the great risk for just a couple of five-minute periods of smoking again? Think about this (silly-sounding, yet profound) statement: The only way to be sure you'll never be a smoker again is to never smoke again.

44. What about your self-image?

Perhaps you are someone who tends to rebel at the thought of accepting the prohibition that you can never smoke again. After all, isn't a person weak indeed if he can't ever let himself touch one more cigarette for fear it will get the best of him? I had been bothered by this when I managed to stay off for a while. What was I saying about me as a person to say I wasn't free to take one little cigarette? In fact, this concern over free will and self-image sent me back to smoking more than once before I finally got off for good.

It was then that it dawned on me that the freedom to be able to smoke occasionally was nothing at all compared to the freedom of being a non-smoker. Non-smokers don't have to check their supplies every time they leave home, don't run like cattle to the street during every intermission and don't find scrounge for butts when they run out of cigarettes. Freedom comes in *not needing* to smoke; it isn't lost in *needing not* to smoke.

45. Do you have freedom?

You have all the freedom in the world, once your cravings end. You will always be free to go back to smoking if you choose, and to stay off if you choose. But please, make a conscious, aware decision. Don't trick yourself with the "just one cigarette" myth. You owe it to yourself to be honest with yourself. If you do go back to smoking, do it because you chose to, not because you unwittingly slipped back into it. You know too much for that to happen now.

About the Author

Joel Block, Ph.D. is a clinical psychologist practicing psychotherapy in New York. He is a senior psychologist on the staff of the North Shore-Long Island Jewish Health System. Dr. Block is also on the clinical faculty (psychiatry/psychology) of the Hofstra University/North Shore-LIJ School of Medicine and he has two board certifications issued by the American Board of Professional Psychology. Dr. Block is a Fellow of the American Psychological Association and the author of over twenty books. He was on the team that researched the Smoke Cessation program used by the American Cancer Society.

I would like to thank the many courageous patients who I have assisted in their smoke cessation quest and who have helped me gain and refine my knowledge of smoke cessation, without which this manual would not have been possible.

Joel Block, Ph.D., ABPP
www.DrBlock.com